The Complete Electric Pressure Cooker Cookbook

Easy and Tasty Recipes that Are Low in Calories

Maria Marshal

Table Of Contents

BREAKFAST RECIPES

Date and Walnut Bread Pudding

(Ready in about 45 minutes | Servings 8)

Ingredients

1. 5 cups stale bread chunks

1. 1 cup dates, pitted and chopped

1. 1/3 cup walnuts, chopped

1. 5 whole eggs

1. 2 cups whole milk

1. 1/4 cup honey

1. 3 tablespoons butter, melted

1. 1 tablespoon flour

1. 1/42 teaspoon ground cinnamon

1. 1/2 teaspoon almond extract

Directions

1. Brush your cake pans with non-stick cooking spray. Toss together breadchunks, dates and walnuts, and drop them into the pans.

2. In a bowl, combine together the remaining ingredients; add the mixture tothe pans. Let it soak for about 10 minutes.

3. Place a trivet at the bottom of your pressure cooker. Then, pour in 2 cups ofwater. Cover the pans with a foil and place them on the trivet.

4. Set the cooker to HIGH for 25 minutes. Serve warm or at room temperature.

Banana and Cranberry Croissant Pudding

(Ready in about 45 minutes | Servings 8)

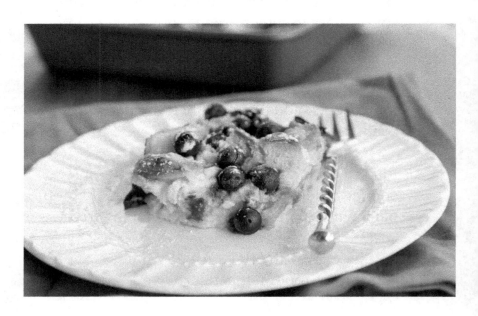

Ingredients

1. 6 cups croissants, torn into pieces

1. 1/2 cup dried bananas, chopped

1. 1/2 cup dried cranberries

1. 5 large eggs

1. 1 ½ cups milk

1. 1/2 cup heavy cream

1. 1/2 cup sugar

1. 2 tablespoons butter, melted

1. 1/4 teaspoon grated nutmeg

1. 1/2 teaspoon ground cinnamon

Directions

1. Brush a soufflé dish with non-stick cooking spray.

2. In a bowl, combine together torn croissants, dried bananas, and cranberries;toss to combine. Then, add this croissants mixture to the soufflé dish.

3. In a bowl, combine together the remaining ingredients; stir to combine. Letit soak for 10 minutes.

4. Lay a trivet at the bottom of a cooker. Pour 2 cups of water to create a waterbath. Cover the dish with a foil, and place on trivet in the cooker. Bring to HIGH pressure and cook for 25 minutes.

5. Release pressure and allow your pudding to rest for 10 minutes beforeserving.

Healthy Strawberry Jam

(Ready in about 1 hour 20 minutes |
Servings 16)

Ingredients

1. 2 pounds strawberries, hulled and halved

1. 1 vanilla bean, halved lengthwise

1. 1 ½ pounds honey

Directions

1. Put all the above ingredients into the pressure cooker. Then, place the uncovered cooker over medium-high heat, bringing it to a boil; make sureto stir frequently.

2. Now lock the cooker's lid into place and bring it to pressure. After that,lower the heat to medium-low for 10 minutes. Take your pressure cookeroff the heat; allow pressure to release naturally.

3. Uncover the cooker and place it back on medium-high heat; bring to a boilfor about 4 minutes, stirring constantly.

4. Spoon the jam into hot sterilized jars. Seal the jars properly. Serve withyour favorite biscuits. Enjoy!

Breakfast Dessert Oatmeal

(Ready in about 15 minutes | Servings 2)

Ingredients

1. 3/4 cup water

1. 1 cup coconut milk

1. 1 cup quick-cooking oats

1. 2 pears, peeled, cored, and diced

1. 1/2 teaspoon vanilla essence

1. 1/2 teaspoon cardamom

1. 1 teaspoon ground cinnamon

1. 2 tablespoons almonds, chopped

Directions

1. Put all of the above ingredients into your pressure cooker. Now lock the lid.Bring to HIGH pressure and maintain for 5 to 6 minutes.

2. Remove the cooker from the heat; allow pressure to release gradually.

3. Serve with some extra milk if desired.

Banana Pecan Oatmeal

(Ready in about 10 minutes | Servings 2)

Ingredients

1. 3⁄4 cup water

1. 1 cup soymilk

1. 1 cup toasted quick-cooking oats

1. 2 bananas, sliced

1. 1/4 cup golden raisins

1. 2 tablespoons honey

1. 2 teaspoons cinnamon

1. 2 tablespoons pecans, chopped

Directions

1. Drop all of the ingredients into the cooker.

2. Lock the lid. Bring it to HIGH pressure and maintain for about 5 minutes. Remove from the heat and bring pressure down

3. Uncover and stir the mixture. Serve with some extra dried fruits or milk ifdesired.

FAST SNACKS RECIPES
Amazing Red Potatoes
(Ready in about 10 minutes | Servings 12)

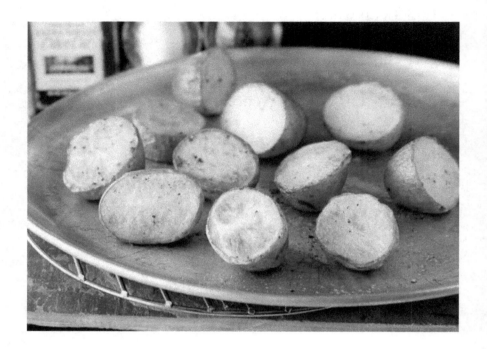

Ingredients

1. 1 cup water

1. 1 teaspoon vegetable oil

1. 3 pounds whole and unpeeled red potatoes, washed and cubed

1. Salt and black pepper, to taste

1. Paprika, to taste

Directions

1. Put the water and vegetable oil into your pressure cooker. Place a rack inyour cooker; load the cooker with potato cubes.

2. Close the lid and bring to pressure over HIGH heat. Cook for 3 minutes;turn off the heat; use quick release method to depressurize your cooker.

3. Season prepared potatoes with salt, black pepper, and paprika. Enjoy!

Party Eggplant Dip

(Ready in about 10 minutes | Servings 12)

Ingredients

1. 1 tablespoon sesame oil

1. 3 cloves garlic, minced

1. 1 large eggplant, peeled and diced

1. 1/2 cup water

1. 3 tablespoons fresh cilantro

1. 1/2 teaspoon salt

1. 1/4 teaspoon ground black pepper

1. 2 tablespoons fresh lemon juice

1. 2 tablespoons tahini

1. 1 tablespoon extra-virgin olive oil

Directions

1. Warm the sesame oil in the pressure cooker over medium heat. Add garlicand eggplant and sauté until they begin to get soft. Pour in the water.

20

2. Lock the cooker's lid and bring to HIGH pressure. Now maintain pressurefor 4 minutes. After that, quick release the pressure and remove the lid.

3. Pulse the eggplant-garlic mixture in your food processor along with thecilantro, salt, black pepper, lemon juice, and tahini.

4. Then, pour in the extra-virgin olive oil and process until the mixture issmooth. Garnish with fresh chopped chives if desired and serve.

Stuffed Potato Shells

(Ready in about 40 minutes | Servings 6)

Ingredients

1. 2 cups water

1. 6 Idaho potatoes, washed

1. 2 tablespoons olive oil

1. 1/4 cup bacon bits

1. 1 cup Cheddar cheese, shredded

1. 1 teaspoon garlic powder

1. 1 teaspoon onion powder

1. 1/4 cup sour cream

Directions

1. Preheat your oven to 400 degrees F. Pour the water into your pressurecooker.

2. Slice the potatoes in half lengthwise. Place the steamer basket in the cooker. Then, arrange the potatoes in two layers in the steamer basket.

3. Then, lock the lid into place. Bring to HIGH pressure and cook for 10 minutes. Next, quick-release the pressure, and uncover the cooker. Then,scoop out the inside of the potatoes, leaving 1/4-thick shells.

4. Grease the scooped-out shell of each potato with olive oil. Layer them on abaking sheet. Bake them for 15 minutes; remove from the oven.

5. Stuff prepared potato skins with the bacon bits and cheese. Sprinkle withgarlic powder and onion powder; then, bake for 10 minutes longer. Servewith sour cream.

LUNCH RECIPES
Chicken Soup with Farfalle

(Ready in about 25 minutes | Servings 6)

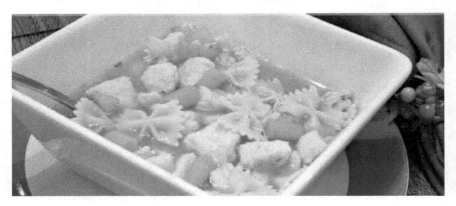

Ingredients

1. 1 pound chicken breasts, boneless, skinless and cubed

1. 2 tablespoons flour

1. Salt and ground black pepper, to taste

1. 3 tablespoons butter

1. 1 onion, diced

1. 2 large-sized carrots, sliced

1. 3 large-sized celery ribs, sliced

1. 1 ½ cups uncooked farfalle pasta

1. 6 cups chicken stock

1. 3/4 teaspoon salt

1. 1/2 teaspoon black pepper

1. 1/2 teaspoon cayenne pepper

1. 1 cup frozen corn kernels, thawed

Directions

1. Toss the chicken cubes with flour; generously season with salt and groundblack pepper.

2. Then, warm the butter on HIGH until melted and sizzling.

3. Lay the coated chicken at the bottom of your pressure cooker; cook forabout 5 minutes or until lightly browned, turning once.

4. Add the onion, carrots, and celery. Top with farfalle pasta and chicken stock; season with salt, black pepper, and cayenne pepper. Seal the lid andcook for 6 minutes on HIGH.

5. Now, release the cooker's pressure. Afterwards, stir in corn kernels andsimmer

for 1 to 2 minutes. Serve warm.

Creamed Tomato Soup

(Ready in about 20 minutes | Servings 6)

Ingredients

1. 2 tablespoons butter

1. 1 onion, diced

1. 1 (28-ounce) can tomato sauce

1. 4 cups chicken broth

1. 8 tomatoes, finely chopped

1. 2 cloves garlic, minced

1. 1/2 teaspoon basil

1. 1/2 teaspoon oregano

1. Sea salt and ground black pepper, to taste

1. 1 cup heavy cream

Directions

1. Warm the butter on HIGH until melted.

2. Cook the onion in the pressure cooker for about 5 minutes.

3. Add the remaining ingredients, except for heavy cream. Seal the lid andcook for 8 minutes on HIGH.

4. Let the pressure release naturally for 5 to 10 minutes. Serve topped withheavy cream.

Soup with Cheese Tortellini

(Ready in about 15 minutes | Servings 6)

Ingredients

1. 2 tablespoons canola oil

1. 2 garlic cloves, minced

1. 1 onion, diced

1. 2 carrots, sliced

1. 2 stalks celery, cut into 1/4 inch slices

1. 1 cup dry cheese tortellini

1. 4 cups vegetable stock

1. 1 (24-ounce) jar spaghetti sauce

1. 1 (14.5-ounce) can diced tomatoes

1. Sea salt and ground black pepper

Directions

1. Heat canola oil in your pressure cooker over HIGH heat.

2. Sauté the garlic, onion, carrots, and celery until tender.

3. Add the rest of the ingredients; stir to combine. Now lock the lid, set thepressure cooker to HIGH and cook for about 5 minutes.

4. Serve topped with grated Cheddar cheese if desired.

DINNER RECIPES
Red Cabbage with Pine Nuts

(Ready in about 10 minutes | Servings 8)

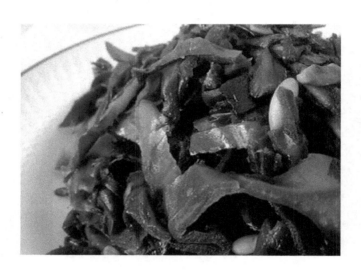

Ingredients

1. 2 tablespoons olive oil

1. 1 onion, diced

1. 2 apples, peeled, cored, and sliced

1. 1/2 cup white wine

1. 1 head red cabbage, cut into strips

1. 1 teaspoon kosher salt

1. 1/2 teaspoon freshly ground black pepper

1. Pine nuts, for garnish

Directions

1. Heat olive oil in your pressure cooker over medium heat. Sauté the onionuntil translucent and soft.

2. Add the apples and wine.

3. Stir the cabbage into the pressure cooker. Cover and cook for 2 to 4 minutesat HIGH pressure.

4. When time is up, open the pressure cooker according to manufacturer's instructions. Season with salt and black pepper. Sprinkle with pine nuts andserve immediately.

Delicious Carrots in Milk Sauce

(Ready in about 10 minutes | Servings 4)

Ingredients

1. 1 pound carrots, cut into 1-inch chunks

1. 1/4 cup water

1. 3/4 cup milk

1. Sea salt and white pepper, to taste

1. 2 tablespoons olive oil

1. 1 tablespoon flour

Directions

1. Fill your cooker with carrots, water, milk, salt, white pepper, and olive oil.Cover with the lid.

2. Turn the heat up to HIGH. Cook approximately 4 minutes at HIGH pressure. Afterwards, open the pressure cooker by releasing pressure.

3. Next, remove carrots to serving dish using a slotted spoon.

4. To make the sauce: Place the pressure cooker over medium heat. Add flourand cook until the sauce has thickened, stirring continuously. Serve the sauce over prepared carrots and enjoy!

Flavorful Ginger Carrots

(Ready in about 5 minutes | Servings 4)

Ingredients

1. 1 pound carrots, peeled and cut into matchsticks

1. 2 tablespoons olive oil

1. 1 teaspoon fresh ginger, minced

1. 1 cup water

1. Kosher salt and ground black pepper, to your taste

1. 1/2 teaspoon allspice

Directions

1. Add the carrot matchsticks, olive oil, ginger, and water to your cooker. Stir to combine well. Close and lock the cooker's lid.

2. Cook for 1 minute at HIGH pressure. Open the pressure cooker according to manufacturer's directions.

3. Season with salt, black pepper and allspice; serve right away!

Butter Corn Evening Treat

(Ready in about 10 minutes | Servings 4)

Ingredients

1. 4 ears sweet corn, shucked

1. 1/2 cup water

1. 1 tablespoon butter

1. 1/2 teaspoon cinnamon

1. Salt and white pepper, to taste

Directions

1. Place a rack in your pressure cooker; arrange the corn on the rack. Pour inthe water.

2. Then, bring to LOW pressure; maintain pressure for about 3 minutes.Remove the lid according to manufacturer's directions.

3. Spread softened butter over each ear of corn; sprinkle with cinnamon, saltand white pepper. Serve.

DESSERT RECIPES
Coconut and Date Rice Pudding
(Ready in about 10 minutes | Servings 6)

Ingredients

1. 2 tablespoons butter

1. 1 cup rice

1. 2 cups water

1. 1/2 teaspoon ground cinnamon

1. 2 cups almond milk

1. 1 cup coconut, shredded

1. 1/2 cup fresh dates, pitted and chopped

1. 1/3 cup sugar

1. Mini chocolate chips, for garnish

Directions

1. Warm the butter in your pressure cooker over medium-high heat. Add the rice and sauté for 1 minute.

2. Add the water and ground cinnamon.
    Cover the cooker and set for 6 minutes
    on HIGH.

3. Then, perform a quick release to release the
    pressure.

4. Add the remaining ingredients. Stir to
    combine; while the pudding is stillhot,
    garnish with chocolate chips.

Spicy Blackberry Sauce

(Ready in about 15 minutes | Servings 8)

Ingredients

1. 2 cups frozen blackberries

1. 2/3 cup grape juice

1. 1/2 cup water

1. 1/8 teaspoon grated nutmeg

1. 1/4 teaspoon cardamom

1. 1/4 teaspoon ground cinnamon

1. 1/2 cup sugar

1. 1 teaspoon vanilla extract

1. 1 tablespoon cornstarch, mixed with 2 tablespoons water

Directions

1. Throw blackberries, grape juice, water, nutmeg, cardamom, and cinnamon in your cooker. Cook for 7 minutes on LOW.

2. Use a quick-release to release the cooker's pressure.

3. Next, use a potato masher to mash the blackberries in the cooker until themixture is nearly puréed.

4. Set the cooker to HIGH, and stir in sugar, vanilla, and cornstarch mixture.Then, simmer the mixture for 3 minutes more.

5. Serve over pancakes or waffles. Enjoy!

Easy Mango Shortcakes

(Ready in about 10 minutes | Servings 8)

Ingredients

1. 3 mangos, peeled and cubed

1. 1/4 cup water

1. 1/2 cup pineapple juice

1. 1/3 cup sugar

1. 1/2 teaspoon vanilla essence

1. 1 1/2 tablespoons cornstarch, mixed with 2 tablespoons water

1. Shortcakes

Directions

1. Place mangos, water, pineapple juice, sugar, and vanilla extract in yourpressure cooker.

2. Cook for 2 minutes on HIGH. Perform a quick release to release thepressure.

3. Then, set the cooker to HIGH and stir in cornstarch mixture; allow tosimmer for 2 minutes, or just until the mixture has thickened.

4. Spoon mango sauce over shortcakes. Serve dolloped with whipped cream ifdesired.

Rice Pudding with Dried Figs

(Ready in about 40 minutes | Servings 8)

Ingredients

1. 1 cup rice

1. 1 ½ cups water

1. A pinch of salt

1. 2 cups whole milk, divided

1. 1/2 cup sugar

1. A dash of cinnamon

1. 2 eggs

1. 1/2 teaspoon vanilla extract

1. 3/4 cup dried figs, chopped

Directions

1. In your pressure cooking pot, combine rice, water, and salt. Place the lid on and select HIGH pressure and 3 minutes cook time. Remove from heat andallow pressure to release naturally.

2. Add 1 ½ cups of milk, sugar and cinnamon to the rice mixture in pressurecooking pot; stir to combine well.

3. In a small-sized bowl, whisk the eggs, remaining 1/2 cup of milk, andvanilla extract. Add to the cooker and cook until mixture begins to boil;make sure to stir frequently. Turn off your cooker.

4. Stir in dried figs. Served dolloped with whipped cream if desired. Enjoy!

INSTANT POT

BREAKFAST RECIPES
Creamed Congee with Strawberries
(Ready in about 45 minutes | Servings 6)

Ingredients

1. 1/2 cup brown rice

1. 1 tablespoon butter

1. 1 teaspoon vanilla extract

1. 1 teaspoon cinnamon powder

1. 1/4 cup dried strawberries, chopped

1. 1 tablespoon honey

1. 7 cups of water

Directions

1. Throw all the above ingredients into your Instant Pot.

2. Choose "Congee" button. Serve at room temperature.

Steamed Eggs with Scallions

(Ready in about 15 minutes | Servings 2)

Ingredients

1. 2 eggs

1. 2/3 cup cold water

1. 1/4 cup scallions, chopped

1. 1 clove garlic, minced

1. Salt and white pepper, to taste

Directions

1. Whisk together the eggs and water in a small-sized mixing bowl. Transferthe mixture to a heat-proof bowl. Add the remaining ingredients; mix tocombine and set aside.

2. Pour 1 cup of water into the inner pot of your Instant Pot. Place the trivet inthe cooker. Place the bowl in the steamer basket.

3. Close the lid and close the vent valve. Press "Manual" setting on HIGH; cook for 5 minutes. Now manually release pressure by turning the valve to'open'. Serve with your favorite bread and enjoy.

47

Eggs with Bacon and Cheese
(Ready in about 25 minutes | Servings 6)

Ingredients

1. 6 medium-sized eggs

1. 1/2 cup heavy cream

1. 1 small-sized leek, finely chopped

1. 1 cup bacon, chopped

1. 1 cup spinach leaves, chopped

1. 1 cup Monterey Jack cheese, shredded

1. Sea salt and ground black pepper, to taste

1. 1/2 teaspoon dried thyme

1. 1/2 teaspoon dried basil

1. 1/4 teaspoon dried oregano

1. Fresh chopped chives, for garnish

Directions

1. In a bowl, whisk the eggs with heavy cream. Add the remaining ingredients, except for chives; mix well to combine.

2. Pour the egg mixture into a heat-proof dish; cover with a foil.

3. Pour 1 cup of water into your cooker. Place the trivet inside. Set the bowlon the trivet. Close the lid tightly.

4. Press "Manual" and HIGH pressure; cook for 20 minutes. Allow thepressure to release naturally. Serve topped with fresh chives.

Ham and Cheese Omelet

(Ready in about 25 minutes | Servings 6)

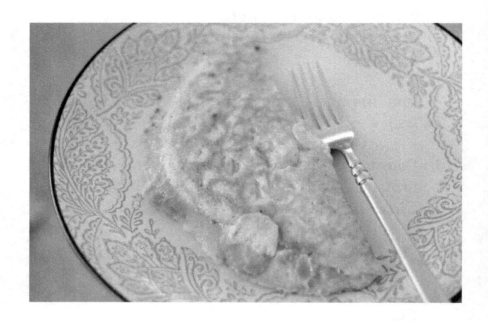

Ingredients

1. 1/2 cup whole milk

1. 6 medium-sized eggs

1. 1 small-sized yellow onion, finely chopped

1. 2 cloves garlic, peeled and minced

1. 1 cup cooked ham, chopped

1. 1 red bell pepper, seeded and thinly sliced

1. 1 handful Cheddar cheese, grated

1. Salt and black pepper, to taste

1. A dash of grated nutmeg

1. 1/2 teaspoon dried basil

Directions

1. Start by whisking the milk and eggs. Add the rest of the above ingredients;stir until everything is well incorporated.

2. Pour this mixture into a heat-resistant dish and cover.

3. Pour 1 cup of water into the base of Instant Pot. Lay the trivet inside. Laythe dish on the trivet.

4. Close the lid. Press "Manual"; cook for 20 minutes under HIGH pressure.Serve right away.

LUNCH RECIPES
Short Ribs with Mushrooms
(Ready in about 50 minutes | Servings 8)

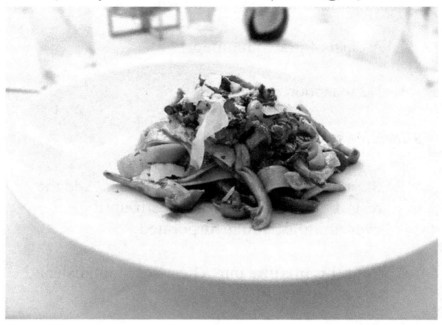

Ingredients

1. 10 short ribs, excess fat trimmed

1. 1 teaspoon salt

1. 3/4 teaspoon ground black pepper

1. 2 tablespoons olive oil

1. 1 cup mushrooms, quartered

1. 1 yellow onion, peeled and chopped

1. 2 carrots, peeled and thinly sliced

1. 2 cloves garlic, peeled and finely minced

1. 2 cups vegetable stock

1. 2 tablespoons tomato ketchup

1. 1 sprig rosemary

Directions

1. First, season the short ribs with salt and ground black pepper. Then, heat olive oil in the inner pot. Choose the "MEAT" function and brown your short ribs on all sides. Set the ribs aside.

2. Add the mushrooms, onion, carrots, and garlic to the pot; then, sauté for 4 minutes.

3. Next, add the ribs back to the pot along with the rest of the ingredients. Now choose the "STEW" function; cook approximately 40 minutes.

4. Transfer to a serving platter and enjoy!

Comforting Potato and Bacon Soup

(Ready in about 20 minutes | Servings 6)

Ingredients

1. 1 yellow onion, peeled and diced

1. 3 slices bacon

1. 1 teaspoon olive oil

1. 2 cups vegetable broth

1. 2 ½ pounds potatoes, peeled and cubed

1. 2 carrots, diced

1. 1 teaspoon cayenne pepper

1. 1 teaspoon dried basil

1. 1/2 teaspoon dried oregano

1. 1/2 teaspoon dried dill weed

1. 1 teaspoon garlic powder

1. 1 cup water

1. 1 ½ cups canned evaporated milk

1. 1 tablespoon salt

1. 3/4 teaspoon ground black pepper

Directions

1. Press "Sauté" function and stir in the onion, bacon, and olive oil. Sauté forabout 4 minutes, stirring continuously.

2. Add vegetable broth, potatoes, carrots, and seasonings. Stir to combine. Cover with the lid, press "Steam" button and adjust the timer to 10 minutes.

3. When beeps, perform a quick pressure release. Remove bacon and reserve.Add water, evaporated milk, salt, and black pepper.

4. Mix with your immersion blender, but leave chunks of potatoes. Taste andadjust the seasonings. Serve with reserved bacon.

Chili Bean Soup

(Ready in about 45 minutes | Servings 6)

Ingredients

1. 1 cup dry beans, soaked in water overnight

1. 1 ham bone

1. 1 bay leaf

1. 1 red onion chopped

1. 1 (15-ounce) can tomatoes, diced

1. 1 celery rib, diced

1. 3 carrots, diced

1. 1 teaspoon chili powder

1. 1 teaspoon cumin powder

1. 1 teaspoon garlic powder

1. Kosher salt and ground black pepper, to taste

Directions

1. Drain and rinse your beans.

2. Put the beans along with ham bone and bay leaf into your cooker; now addjust enough water to cover. Seal Instant Pot and cook on "Bean/Chili" setting.

3. Discard the ham bone and bay leaf; now add remaining ingredients and stirto combine well.

4. Choose "Soup" setting, adjusted down to 20 minutes. Open your potaccording to manufacturer's directions. Serve and enjoy!

Country Chicken and Vegetable Soup

(Ready in about 35 minutes | Servings 6)

Ingredients

1. 2 frozen chicken breasts, boneless and skinless

1. 3 carrots, trimmed and chopped

1. 4 potatoes, diced

1. 1 onion, peeled and diced

1. 4 cups chicken stock

1. Salt and cracked black pepper, to taste

Directions

1. Simply throw all the above ingredients in your Instant Pot.

2. Turn "Manual" setting on your Instant Pot; set the timer for 35 minutes.Serve right away!

DINNER RECIPES
Saucy Salmon Fillets
(Ready in about 10 minutes | Servings 16)

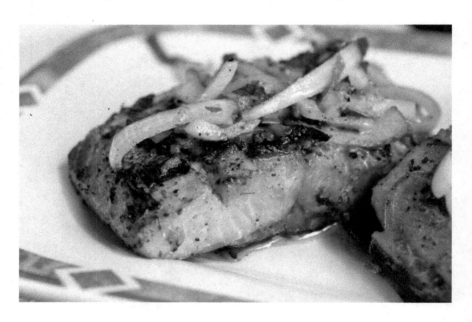

Ingredients

1. 4 salmon filets

1. Salt and ground black pepper, to taste

1. 1 tablespoon lemon juice

1. 3 tablespoons mayonnaise

1. 1 tablespoon brown sugar

1. 2 tablespoons olive oil

1. 1 tablespoon fresh parsley

Directions

1. Season salmon filets with salt and black pepper. Press "Sauté" and brownyour filets on both sides.

2. Add about 3/4 cup water to pot. Lay browned salmon on a rack. Seal thecooker's lid and choose "Steam" for about 5 minutes.

3. In the meantime, mix remaining ingredients in a bowl or a measuring cup.Then, pour the sauce over the filets.

Pork Ribs with Vegetables

(Ready in about 40 minutes | Servings 4)

Ingredients

1. 2 pork ribs

1. 2 cups BBQ sauce

1. 1 cup water

1. 2 onions, slice into rings

1. 2 parsnips, thinly sliced

1. 2 carrots, thinly sliced

Directions

1. Lay the ribs in your Instant Pot. Pour in 1 cup of BBQ sauce and 1 cup ofwater. Close the cooker's lid.

2. Then, press "Meat" key. Add the onions, parsnips, and carrots. Cover withthe lid and choose "Manual" button, and set to 2 minutes. Drizzle with remaining BBQ sauce and serve right now.

Grandma's Juicy Spareribs

(Ready in about 45 minutes | Servings 6)

Ingredients

1. 1 tablespoon olive oil

1. 1 onion, sliced

1. 1/4 cup tomato paste

1. 1/4 tamari sauce

1. 2 tablespoons brown sugar

1. 1/3 cup rice wine vinegar

1. 1 (20-ounce) can of pineapple

1. 1 teaspoon ginger, finely chopped

1. 1 teaspoon granulated garlic

1. 1 teaspoon coriander, ground

1. Salt and black pepper, to taste

1. 4 pounds ribs, cut for serving.

1. Cornstarch slurry

Directions

1. Heat the oil, and sauté the onions until just tender.

2. Stir in the rest of the ingredients, except for cornstarch slurry.

3. Next, choose "Stew" function for 12 minutes. Then, release pressure. Addcornstarch slurry and stir until the juice has thickened. Serve warm and enjoy!

Summer Brown
Rice Salad

(Ready in about 30 minutes | Servings 4)

Ingredients

1. 2 cups brown rice

1. 2 ½ cups water

1. 8 grape tomatoes, halved

1. 1 cucumber, cored and diced

1. 2 bell peppers, sliced

1. 1 cup scallions, chopped

1. 1 teaspoon red pepper flakes

1. Salt and white pepper, to your liking

Directions

1. Add rice and water to your Instant Pot. Close and lock the lid. Press"Manual"; choose 22 minutes pressure cooking time.

2. Next, open the cooker using Natural Pressure Release. Transfer to a bowl inorder to cool completely.

3. Add the rest of the ingredients. Afterwards, gently stir to combine and serve.

Black Bean and Mint Salad

(Ready in about 15 minutes | Servings 4)

Ingredients

1. 1 cup black beans, soaked overnight

1. 4 cups water

1. 3 garlic cloves, smashed

1. 1 sprig fresh mint

1. 1 tablespoon extra-virgin olive oil

1. 1 tablespoon red wine vinegar

1. Salt and freshly cracked black pepper, to your liking

Directions

1. Add black beans, water, and garlic to the inner pot of your Instant Pot.Press "Manual" and choose 8 minutes pressure cooking time.

2. Drain your beans and add the remaining ingredients. Gently stir untileverything is well mixed. Serve chilled and enjoy!

FAST SNACKS
Orange Glazed Sugar Snap and Peas Carrots

(Ready in about 10 minutes | Servings 8)

Ingredients

1. 1 tablespoon butter

1. 1 ½ cups frozen sugar snap peas

1. 1 ½ pounds carrots, cut into matchsticks

1. A pinch of salt

1. White pepper to your liking

1. 3 tablespoons orange marmalade

1. 1/2 teaspoon ground ginger

Directions

1. Simply throw all the ingredients in your Instant Pot.

2. Pressure cook for 4 minutes. Transfer to a serving bowl and serve.

Sausage Dipping Sauce

(Ready in about 15 minutes | Servings 10)

Ingredients

1. 1 tablespoon butter, at room temperature

1. 1/2 pound ground Italian sausage

1. 1 (28-ounce) can crushed tomatoes

1. 1 onion, chopped

1. 2 cloves garlic, sliced

1. 1 teaspoon dried basil

1. 2 tablespoons flour

1. Salt and ground black pepper to taste

Directions

1. Heat the butter in your cooker. Add ground sausage and cook until it isbrowned. Add the remaining ingredients.

2. Close and lock the lid; set the timer to 15 minutes. Release pressurenaturally. Serve with tortilla chips. Enjoy!

Meatballs with Marinara Sauce

(Ready in about 25 minutes | Servings 12)

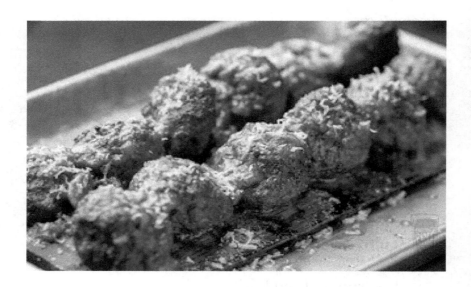

Ingredients

1. 1 tablespoon butter

1. 40 frozen meatballs

1. 2 (16-ounce) jars marinara sauce

1. 1 cup vegetable broth

1. Sea salt and black pepper, to taste

1. 1/4 cup fresh cilantro

Directions

1. Warm the butter in your cooker on "Sauté" setting. Stir in the meatballs andcook until they are browned. Cook for 2 minutes, stirring frequently.

2. Add marinara sauce and vegetable broth. Season with salt and black pepper.Close and lock the lid on your cooker.

3. Set the timer to 20 minutes. Now release the pressure manually. Servesprinkled with fresh cilantro.

Tomato Dipping Sauce

(Ready in about 25 minutes | Servings 12)

Ingredients

1. 1 tablespoon olive oil

1. 3 cloves garlic

1. 1 shallot, chopped

1. 1 parsnip, chopped

1. 1 carrot, chopped

1. 1 teaspoon basil

1. 1 (28-ounce) can crushed tomatoes

1. 1 cup water

1. 1 teaspoon cayenne pepper

1. Salt and black pepper, to taste

1. 1 tablespoon parsley

Directions

1. Click "Sauté" key and warm the olive oil in the cooker. Stir in the garlicand shallot and cook until they are tender, for 1 to 2 minutes.

2. Add the parsnip, carrots, and basil. Pour in the crushed tomatoes and water.

3. Close the lid on the cooker. Set the cooker's timer for 20 minutes. Quickrelease pressure. Season with cayenne pepper, salt, and black pepper.

4. Sprinkle with fresh parsley. Serve with your favorite dippers such as breadsticks or crackers.

DESSERT RECIPES
Bread Pudding with Prunes and Pecans

(Ready in about 30 minutes | Servings 6)

Ingredients

1. 4 cups Ciabatta, cubed

1. 1 teaspoon ghee

1. 1 cup almond milk

1. 1 cup whole milk

1. 3 eggs, beaten

1. 1/2 cup prunes, coarsely chopped

1. 1/4 teaspoon grated nutmeg

1. 1/2 teaspoon cinnamon powder

1. 1/4 teaspoon kosher salt

1. 1 teaspoon vanilla paste

1. Chopped pecans, for garnish

Directions

1. Pour 2 cups of water into the Instant Pot. Place the steam rack at thebottom.

2. Add bread cubes to a casserole dish.

3. In a mixing bowl, combine the remaining ingredients; mix to combine well.Pour this mixture over the bread cubes in the casserole dish. Cover with a wax paper.

4. Set your cooker to "Steam"; adjust the time to 15 minutes. Next, wait anadditional 15 minutes before removing the cooker's lid.

Apricot Oatmeal Dessert

(Ready in about 10 minutes | Servings 4)

Ingredients

1. 4 apricots, pitted and halved

1. 1 cup steel-cut oats

1. 1 cups coconut milk

1. 1/2 teaspoon vanilla paste

1. 2 cups water

1. 1 cup sugar

Directions

1. Stir everything into the inner pot of your cooker. Choose "Manual/Adjust"mode.

2. Set the timer to 3 minutes. Open the lid according to manufacturer'sdirections. Serve garnished with coconut flakes if desired. Enjoy!

Mom's Stuffed Peaches

(Ready in about 15 minutes | Servings 3)

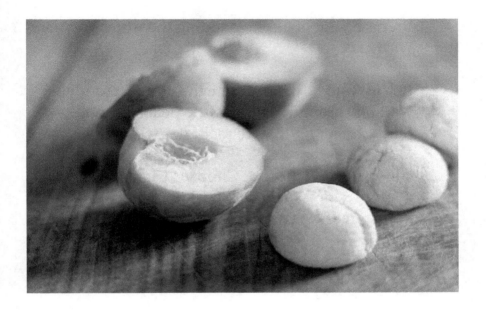

Ingredients

1. 2 cups water

1. 8 cookies, crumbled

1. 2 tablespoons walnuts, chopped

1. 1 teaspoon orange zest

1. 3 peaches, halved and pitted

1. 2 tablespoons butter

Directions

1. Prepare your cooker by adding the water and the wire rack.

2. In a mixing bowl, combine the cookie crumbs, walnuts, orange zest. Stuffthe peaches and place them on the wire rack; dot with butter.

3. Close and lock the lid. Choose "Manual" and 4 minutes pressure cookingtime. Afterwards, quick pressure release. Serve right away.

Baked Apples with Raisins

(Ready in about 15 minutes | Servings 6)

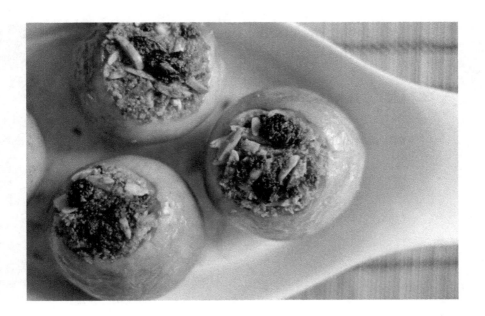

Ingredients

1. 6 apples, cored

1. 1/4 cup raisins

1. 1 cup red wine

1. 1/2 cup brown sugar

1. 1/2 teaspoon grated nutmeg

1. 1 teaspoon cinnamon powder

Directions

1. Lay the apples in the base of your cooker. Add the rest of the ingredients.

2. Cook for 10 minutes at HIGH pressure. Use Natural release method. Dustwith powdered sugar and serve. Enjoy!